Healthy
Fit and Sexy
Your D.I.Y guide to a Size Healthy Lifestyle

Mrs. Nataisha A. Ramirez

ISBN:1497455898
ISBN-13:9781497455894

DEDICATION

I thank my parents for teaching me that as long as I keep God first, all things are possible. I would like to thank my husband, Levi Ramirez Sr. for being there for me through all my ups and downs. I'd like to thank all those who always gave me an encouraging word to keep me going. I dedicate this book to all those suffering with obesity. You are never alone and you will lay aside the weight mentally, physically and spiritually. You just have to believe in yourself, God will do the rest.

CONTENTS

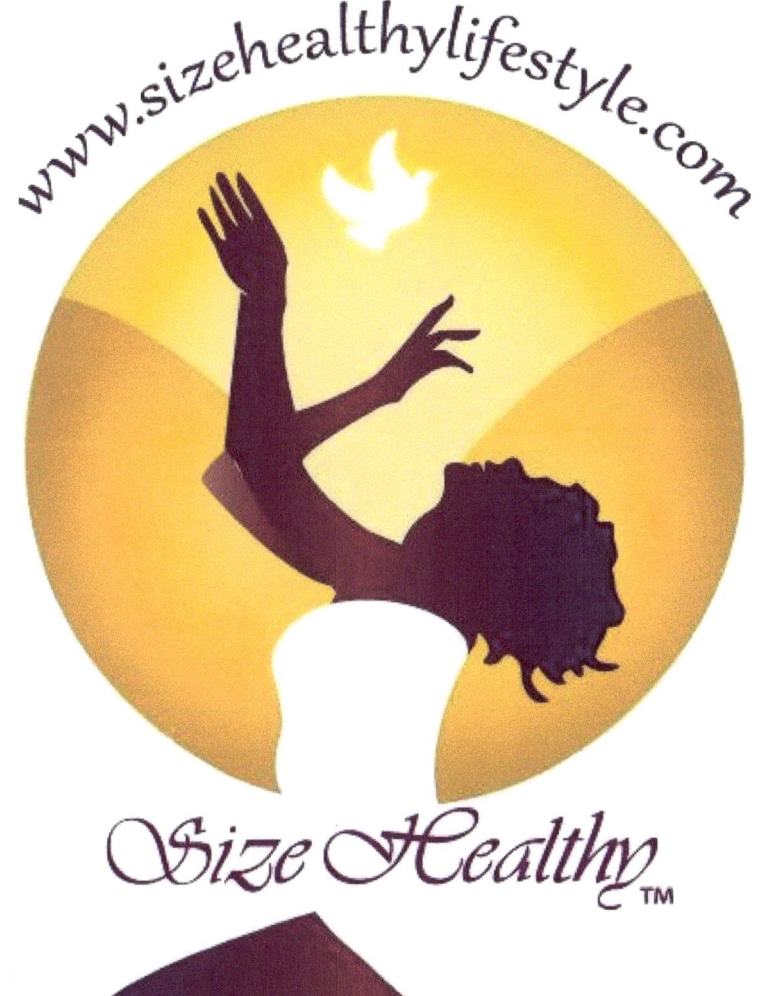

www.sizehealthylifestyle.com

Size Healthy™

Our Mission

Size Healthy is designed to improve the quality of life for women by developing the mind, body, and spirit through physical fitness, education, and a healthy lifestyle change

Size Healthy's Ten Commandments

Thou shall NOT partake in unhealthy foods.
Thou shall NOT worry about what others are doing.
 Thou shall NOT sabotage your thinking with
negative thoughts.
Thou shall NOT compare yourself to others.
Thou shall NOT give up when it gets tough.
Thou shall DO your BEST with what you have.
Thou shall SPEAK positive things about yourself at all times.
Thou shall find the YOUniqueness in what YOU do.
Thou shall Faith it til YOU make it
Thou shall BELIEVE that YOU are strong and capable of being
more and not just good enough!

My name is Nataisha "ADivaRunner" Ramirez and I started Size Healthy because I realized in my struggles, that my thoughts of me were tainted. I wanted to look like everyone else instead of who God created. This epidemic seems to be spreading rapidly throughout the nation amongst women. We desire our bodies to look like someone else's rather than how God created it to look. This is a human reaction that we tend to see with our physical eye; however in the spiritual realm we are more than enough because that is how God made us. He said, that He knew us before we were formed in the womb (Jeremiah 1:5). He knew that we had weaknesses but He has set us apart from everyone else; a YOUnique size designed just for us.

Size Healthy is not a one size fits all program. It is a program designed just for you. You find your YOUniqueness in what you do, which makes your journey original. Size Healthy is not a "diet," it is a healthier way of thinking, eating, and living. This process performs internal surgery that resonates outwardly. This program believes in Godly principles to reach your healthy goals. The first principle that Size Healthy believes in is taking care of the temple. According to 1 Corinthians 3:16-17, "do you know that you are God's temple and that God's spirit dwells in you? If anyone destroys God's temple God will destroy him. For God's temple is holy and you are that temple." You are paying rent to live in a temporary house. Your house must be clean to continue to live there. There are repercussions for not taking care of your house. You will and can be served an eviction notice at any time through diabetes, coronary heart disease, hypertension, obesity, etc. A Size Healthy lifestyle is a change to a healthier you. Size Healthy deals with the mind, body and spirit to tackle the unhealthy choices that you have made. It takes 21 days to form a habit and 90 days to develop a lifestyle change. Are you ready to make a 180 degree change in order to be healthy? This journey is about you. Your size and your health are your choice. You have the ability to choose an alternative way of eating. Some say it costs more to eat healthy and less to eat fast food, but the lower costing foods (i.e. fast foods) cause the most detrimental consequences in your life; death.

If you were to examine your life based off what you were feeding your body; mentally, physically, and spiritually how long would you live? Would you die today or live a life of longevity?

THERE ARE 4 STAGES TO LIVING A SIZE HEALTHY LIFESTYLE.

1. DESIRE
2. DECISION
3. DETERMINATION
4. DISCIPLINE

EACH STAGE IS A PROCESS, WITH STRATEGIES FOR SUCCEEDING AT EVERY LEVEL.

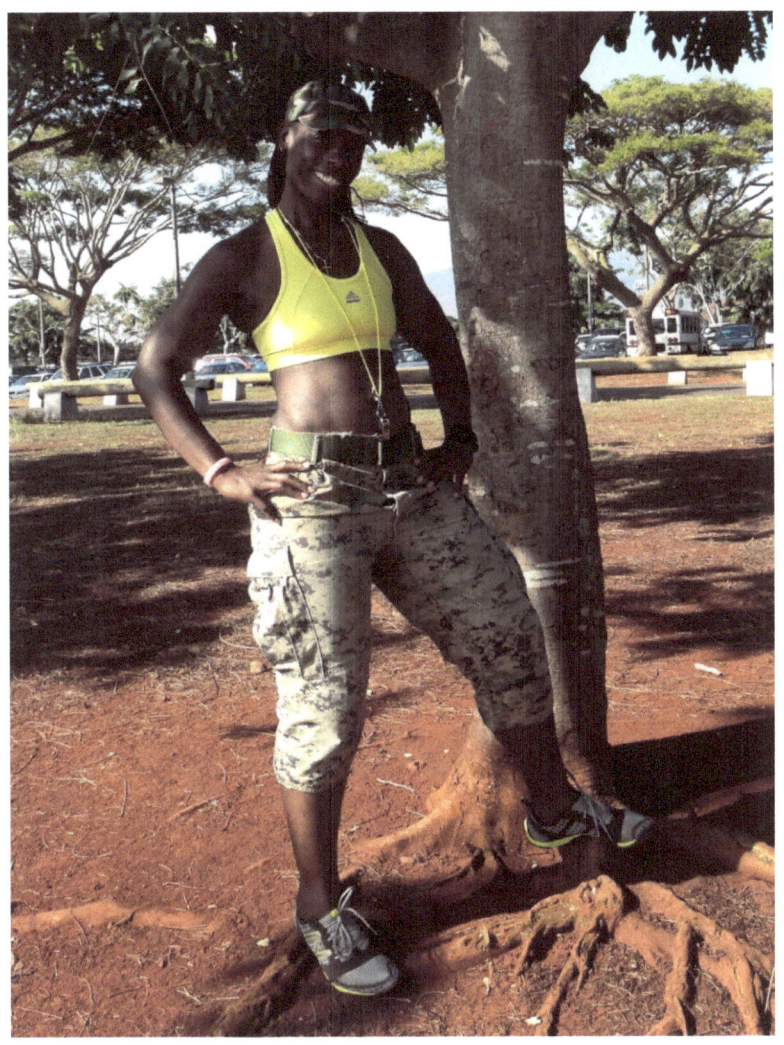

1 DESIRE

The first step is acknowledging that a change has to take place. You are aware of the problem, you are considering a change, but you are leery about being committed to that which you want. You are reminded of how much work it will take and not sure if you are willing to put in the hours. You are aware that change is good for you, but due to the pain that you believe you will encounter you self sabotage. Wanting to change and not wanting to change are normal; however they are also a conflicting state of mind...he is a double-minded man, unstable in all he does (James 1:8). In this stage the statements you make are: *I can't go to a gym until I lose more weight, I need to lose weight but it cost too much to eat healthy, I want to lose weight but I don't know where to begin, I want to lose weight but I have no one to help me, I should stop eating junk but I am stressed out, I want to run but I cannot and the list goes on.*

The BUTS (blaming your thoughts) are arguments or excuses in your mind. You cancel your BUTS by thinking why you should rather than why you should not.. Our desires change from one day to the next, which makes the decision process harder. Most times the only way change will occur is something detrimental happening, such as a diagnosis from your physician or a heart attack/stroke has occurred. Why must we wait until something happens in order for change to occur? As humans, we have to be forced into a decision to change our behavior. You have to change your talk in order to be successful at what you desire. In the desire stage, if you continue to think about changing and wishing you could change but no progress is being made, **YOU ARE NOT READY!**

2 DECISION

Congratulations! You are ready to make a change because you are "sick and tired of being sick and tired." You want to be a healthier version of you. Your talk has changed from wanting and needing, blaming your thoughts (BUT), to *I wish, I want and I like*. This is great because you have intensions of doing what you desire rather than just having a conversation with self. You can do anything you put your mind to. Philippians 4:13 says, " I CAN (control and navigate) do all things through Christ who strengthens me." The will to do is there; however you have to activate it. You will make statements such as *I can, I could, I might be able, I think I can, etc*. When you make a decision to do something we activate an internal motivation that appears outwardly. Sometimes our decisions for change are based off of reasons, which is perfectly okay because that promotes accountability. These statements are: *I am sure if I exercised more I would have more energy, I want to lose weight so that I can see my children grow up, I am sure if I drink more water it would be better for my kidneys, etc*. As humans, we need to do many things, however our thought process is tainted. An example of this... *I should be exercising but I have no time, I want to eat healthy, but healthier food is expensive, I would love to stop drinking soda, but I need the caffeine, etc*.

In the decision process, your desire to change your behavior has been activated. You begin to write out S.M.A.R.T goals: specific, measurable, attainable, reachable, and timely. However, writing them out does not trigger the behavior change alone; doing does. You might waiver during this stage and if so, just get back up and start over. Don't give up because you are not defeated! It will just take a little more time for you to get to your goal.

S.M.A.R.T. Goal example:

In 30 days, I will begin going to the gym in the morning, 3 times a week for 90 minutes each day. I will do cardio for 60 minutes and 30 minutes of strength training. I will stick to this plan for 30 days before changing my routine. It takes 21 days to form a habit and if you continue this routine for more than 21 days, you have developed a habit.

3 DETERMINATION

You are committed! No matter what it feels like, looks like, or taste like you are determined to do this. You have made successful strides towards a healthier you. You have figured it out and realize that it is not as hard as you imagined. You have been successful for 90 days, which is a lifestyle change. You realize that you need this not only for your body, but for peace of mind. You are much happier now. This is not to say that things do not happen, because according to James 1:2, "We are to consider it pure joy, my brothers, whenever you face trials of many kinds, because you know that the testing of your faith develops perseverance." The activation of your faith (fearless acts in the heart) is your determination to keep going. Your determination will without a doubt keep you moving even when you hit a wall. This journey is not easy. According to Romans 12:2, "Do not be conformed any longer to the pattern of this world, but be transformed by the renewing of your mind. Then you will be able to test and approve what God's will is- his good, pleasing and perfect will." There is nothing physical about living a healthy lifestyle. I had to learn this the hard way. Living a healthy lifestyle is a mental journey that resonates in the physical realm. This is why you have tried and failed, failed and tried, and the process goes on and on.

We must change our mind in order for change to occur outwardly. In this phase, you should be mentally trying to find ways to keep a healthy lifestyle. Your journey is not like anyone else's so you must find things that will help you continue this journey or else you will give up. Remember this is not a diet, its a lifestyle change. It is a change into a healthier you. Everyone's healthy does not look the same but it does have the same ingredients; so, do not compare what you do to someone else. Developing new habits requires you to write them down step by step. Put it "YOU" on your "TO DO" list.

Your determination now sounds like this: *I will, I promise, I am ready to, I intend to, I guarantee.*

4 **DISCIPLINE**

You have formed a lifestyle of health. You are pressing through life and no matter what goes on **YOUR HEALTH MATTERS!** You know it can be done and you are now a role model for others. It is still not easy but when things get in the way you know how to overcome obstacles because you have made up in your mind, "**For with God nothing shall be impossible.**" (Luke 1:37)

You have a routine and because you are discipline you make sure that routine is not broken. In this stage you have probably lost some friends along the way because you no longer do the things you use to do, go the places you use to go or talk the way you use to talk. Don't be depressed about it because you can not take everyone with you and not everyone is ready to be healthy. You chose to be a healthier you and although you may want everyone to be healthy too, it just does not work as you may have imagined. So love them from a distance and pray that they too will begin to take their health seriously. Remember those that mind, don't matter and those that matter don't mind.
You have done well with the steps and if you find yourself reverting to old habits just repeat the stages again. Many times we see the goal before we reach it but the process requires you to **BELIEVE** in **YOU**rself and NEVER give up. Gather your thoughts and put them in perspective. Make small goals and stick with them.

Questions to ask yourself:

1. What do I need to do in order to stay committed?

2. How will I stay motivated?

21 Days to a Healthier You

IT TAKES 21 DAYS TO DEVELOP A HABIT. YOU WILL
FEEL LIKE GIVING UP BUT IF YOU STAY THE COURSE
AND WORK THROUGH THE PRESSURE YOU WILL SEE
RESULTS. "THE RACE IS NOT GIVEN TO THE SWIFT BUT
TO THOSE WHO ENDURE TO THE END."
(ECCLESIASTES 9:11)

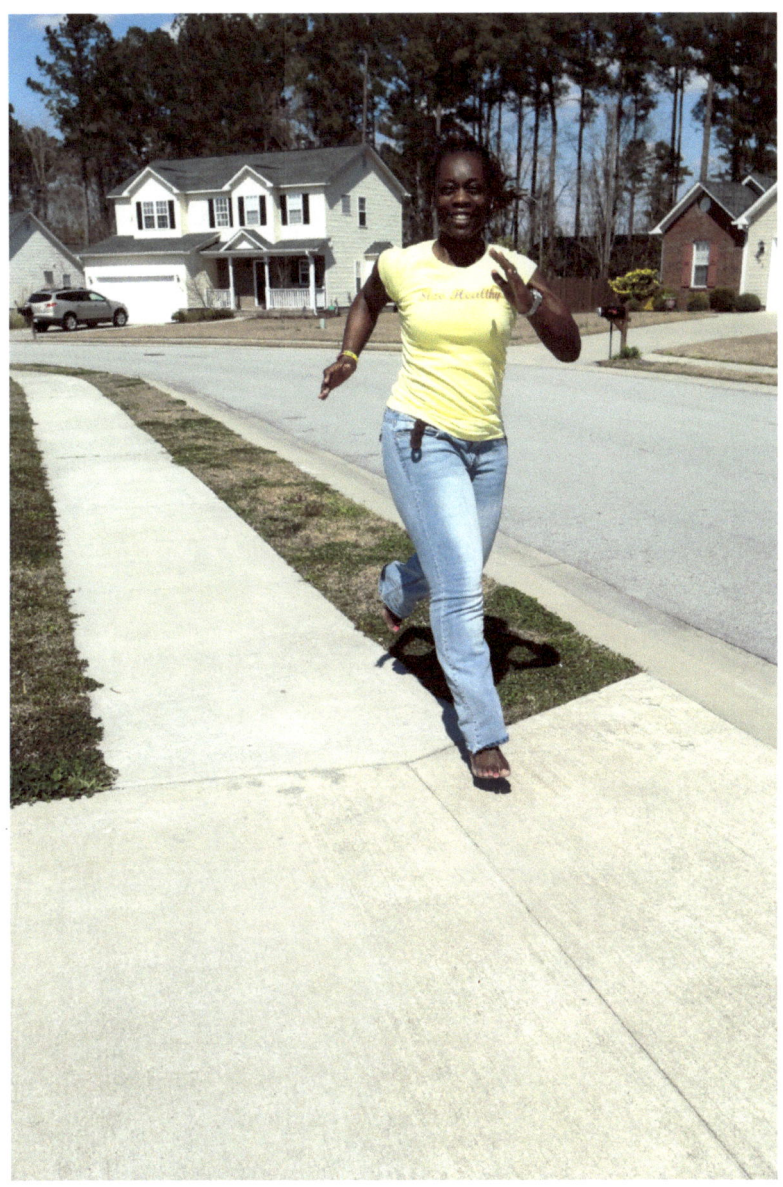

DAY 1

Desire

22"Do not merely listen to the word, and so deceive yourselves. Do what it says. 23 Anyone who listens to the word but does not do what it says is like a man who looks at his face in a mirror 24 and, after looking at himself, goes away and immediately forgets what he looks like." James 1:22-24

You have just sat down to watch television and you see a commercial that shows women in the gym working out. You say to yourself, I want to lose 10 lbs., but as soon as the commercial goes off that thought has quickly gotten lost in space. We all have wants and desires but when we do not act upon them or seek help, they become one way conversations with me, myself, and I. The bible says "Act on what you hear." If you said you need to lose 10 lbs. then act on it. If you can not do it by yourself, seek help.

~ Look at yourself and find the change within.

Journal Notes: What are your desires?

_____

_____

_____

_____

_____

_____

_____

_____

_____

_____

_____

_____

_____

_____

_____

_____

_____

_____

_____

DAY 2

Examine Yourself

"For physical training is of some value, but godliness has value for all things, holding promise for both the present life and the life to come." 1 Tim 4:8

Conversations between me, myself and I continue to get tossed and driven within the mind. You still have not activated your desire to put a plan in place. You are still talking and wishing you could walk a mile, do a sit up, or even run a block. These things will NEVER change as long as your conversation with self continues to be I WISH, I CAN'T, I WOULD, and I COULD. Those words are versions of who you use to be. In order to become the person you desire to be, you must ACTIVATE your FAITH MUSCLES.

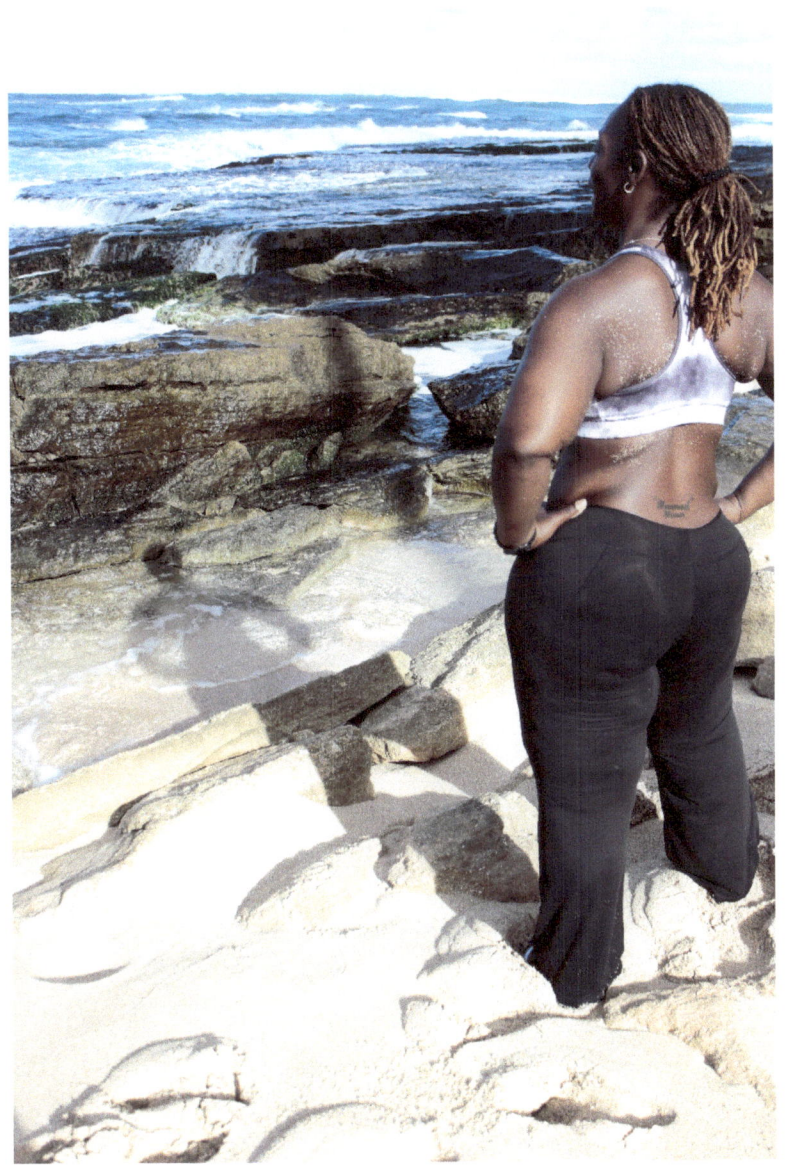

Journal Notes:

What do you see when you look in the mirror?

_____

_____

_____

_____

_____

_____

_____

_____

_____

_____

_____

_____

_____

_____

_____

_____

_____

DAY 3
Stop talking yourself out of it

3"When we put bits into the mouths of horses to make them obey us, we can turn the whole animal. 4 Or take ships as an example. Although they are so large and are driven by strong winds, they are steered by a very small rudder wherever the pilot wants to go. 5 Likewise the tongue is a small part of the body, but it makes great boasts. Consider what a great forest is set on fire by a small spark. 6 The tongue also is a fire, a world of evil among the parts of the body. It corrupts the whole person, sets the whole course of his life on fire, and is itself set on fire by hell." James 3:3-6

I am at the starting line and I am waiting for the gun to go off. I am talking amongst friends and I tell them, " I have never ran a race, nor have I been running so you might leave me because I don't run that fast." You will do fine is what I was told. On your mark, get set, GOooo! The gun goes off and all feet hit the pavement except for mine. I stalled because I had no gas. I slowly walked the entire race while having conversations with me, myself, and I. I desired to run, but didn't practice. The worst thing was that I sabotaged myself with my thoughts of "I have NEVER ran before." Everyone has to start somewhere, so where will you start or will you continue to have bubbles of thoughts that you quickly pop with negativity?

Journal Notes:

What have you talked yourself out of ?

_____

_____

_____

_____

_____

_____

_____

_____

_____

_____

_____

_____

_____

_____

_____

_____

_____

_____

_____

_____

_____

Day 4

Its time to FIGHT!

"For our struggle is not against flesh and blood, but against the rulers, against the authorities, against the powers of this dark world and against the spiritual forces of evil in the heavenly realms." *Ephesians 6:12*

Giants are big and cause stress! This stress overwhelms us, causing us not to be able to function in our daily activities. The only way to fight a giant is to face it head on. I have encountered many giants during my journey and there were times when I allowed the giants to just do as they pleased because I had no fight left in me. I could no longer stand up for myself but the Bible says, "We wrestle not against flesh and blood but against principalities, against powers, against the rulers of the darkness of this age, against spiritual hosts of wickedness in heavenly places" (Ephesians 6:12) We must tap into something deeper than what appears on the surface. Your giants did not just get there or apear out of the sky. You have been dealing with them your entire life and they have caused strife amongst your inner and outer layers of self. It's time to fight and defeat the giant.

~ Turn your BIG G into a little g

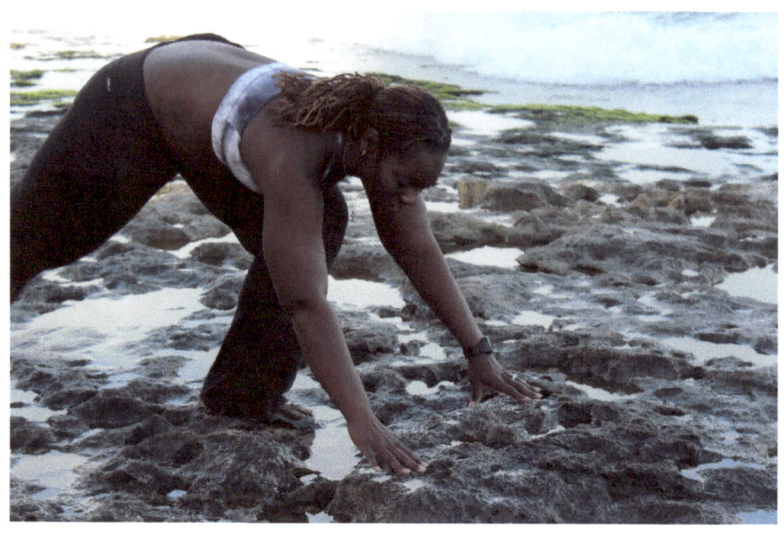

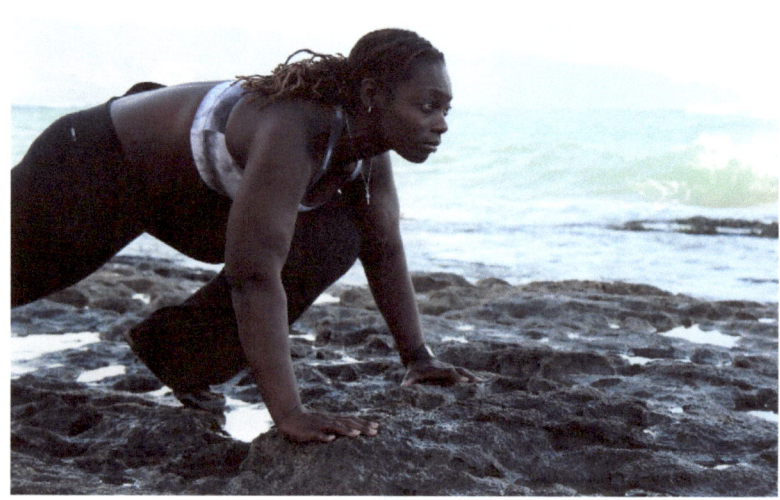

Journal Notes:

David used 5 smooth stones to fight Goliath, what five stones will you use?

1.Who are you?

2.Whose are you?

3. Why were you created (purpose)?

4. What can you do to help yourself?

5. When will you begin?

_____

_____

_____

_____

_____

_____

_____

_____

_____

_____

DAY 5

Know your value

"For the weapons of our warfare are not carnal but mighty in God for pulling down strongholds, casting down arguments and every high thing that exalts itself against the knowledge of God, bringing every thought into captivity to the obedience of Christ." 2 Cor 10: 4-5

"I am not good enough! I can not do it because the more I try, the harder I fall." How do you expect to reach your destination or destiny with desires of negativity. A positive plus a negative doesn't equal a positive unless the positive is greater than the negative; however in math this may be true but life has a way of being far more than that. You do more harm to yourself than the world does, so its time out for thinking I am not good enough because God says you are fearfully and wonderfully made. You were not meant to be like anyone else. Stand out and stop blending in. Find the **YOU** in everything **YOU** do and **YOU** will succeed every time.

~ Don't be a copy version of someone else, be a BEST SELLER!

Journal Notes:

In what ways can you stand out?

_____

_____

_____

_____

_____

_____

_____

_____

_____

_____

_____

_____

_____

_____

_____

_____

_____

_____

_____

_____

Day 6

Moving Forward

20 "Once, having been asked by the Pharisees when the kingdom of God would come, Jesus replied, "The kingdom of God does not come with your careful observation, 21 nor will people say, 'Here it is,' or 'There it is,' because the kingdom of God is within you." Luke 17:20-21

Your house is eroding. The windows and doors have been closed for so long that the smell has a sweet aroma to you and you wonder why you can't get out. You have the power within you to move but fear and your lack of confidence in yourself is holding you back. Can you not smell the infirmities burning inside of you? You have the ability to move but your "woe is me" attitude has locked you behind a close door. However the good news is that you have the key to open the door. No one has to tell you "how" and "when" because its been in you all this time. The key is you and the sooner you unlock the door, the easier it will be.

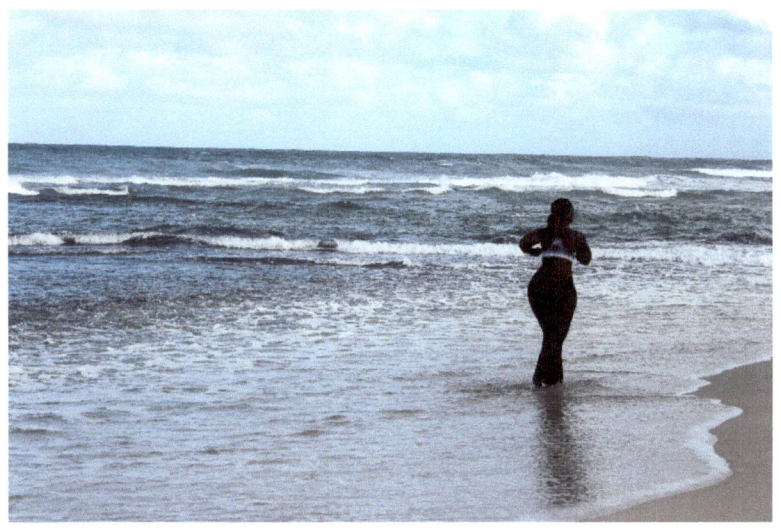

Journal Notes:

What thoughts are you considering but not activating?

_____

_____

_____

_____

_____

_____

_____

_____

_____

_____

_____

_____

_____

_____

_____

_____

_____

_____

_____

_____

_____

DAY 7

Yes, I Can

"I can do everything through him who gives me strength."
Philippians 4:13

Anytime we make a decision to change there is a process that we must follow. The first step is planning. Winston Churchill stated, " He who fails to plan is planning to fail." Don't think because you have made a decision to do it that it will go smoothly. Planning provides strategies to endure. When we plan, we must be smart about it: specific, measurable, achievable, realistic, and timely. Don't have high expectations when you have NEVER exercised or haven't been eating a nutritious meal. We all have to start somewhere so start off small and work you way up. I CAN (control and navigate) all things through Christ who gives me strength.

~ Small steps create BIG changes

Journal Notes:

What is your 21 day plan?

(It takes 21 days to form a habit)

_____

_____

_____

_____

_____

_____

_____

_____

_____

_____

_____

_____

_____

_____

_____

_____

_____

_____

_____

_____

_____

_____

_____

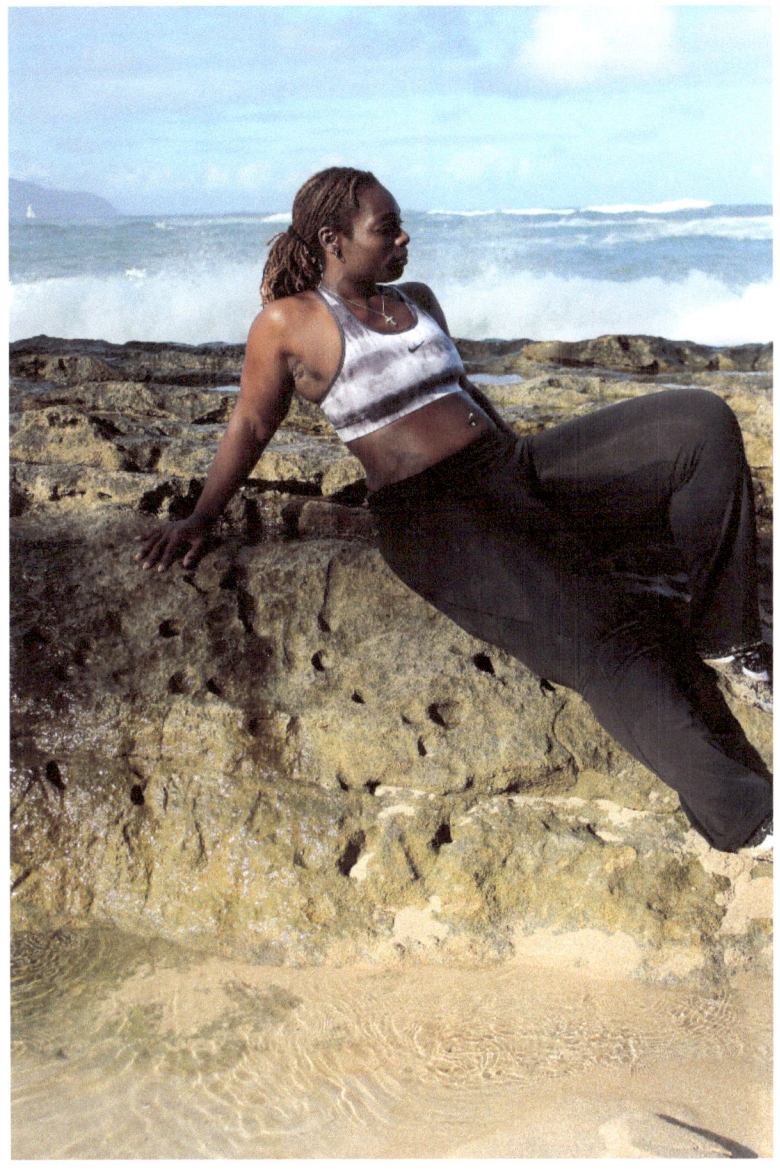

DAY 8

Plan, Prepare, Press!

Things don't always go the way we plan but walking through the door of defeat doesn't make it any easier. Anytime we prepare ourselves for something new the devil will try to open the door of chaos. I want you to press pass that door. Slam it shut and keep climbing. You have what it takes to succeed but don't expect it to be easy.

~ HOW BAD DO YOU WANT IT?

Journal Notes:

What walls have you hit?

_____

_____

_____

_____

_____

_____

_____

_____

_____

_____

_____

_____

_____

_____

_____

_____

_____

_____

_____

_____

_____

DAY 9

What seeds are you sowing?

"The body is a unit, though it is made up of many parts; and though all its parts are many, they form one body. So it is with Christ." 1 Corinthians 12:12

Planning and preparing isn't the job of just one part of the body. Planning and preparing involves your whole being and if one part of the body doesn't do its part the entire body fails. The mind is a powerful part of the body and can help or hinder the planning and preparation process. If you allow your mind to focus on everything that is negative, strongholds begin to consume the mind like a burning flame. However, positive thinking provides hope. Don't allow your mind to sabotage the rest of the body through impure thoughts. Focus on the positives and you will reap a harvest of completion.

Self control is the ability to guide your actions in pursuit of a goal - to persevere and stay on course despite temptations, distractions, and the demands of competing goals.

~ Heidi Halvorson PhD

Journal Notes:

What's special about your seeds?

_____

_____

_____

_____

_____

_____

_____

_____

_____

_____

_____

_____

_____

_____

_____

_____

_____

_____

_____

DAY 10

Got Faith?

"Now faith is being sure of what we hope for and certain of what we do not see." Hebrews 11:1

Faith is fearless acts in the heart. You know that you need to do this for yourself but fear continues to cloud your mind. Fear is a spirit and the longer you allow it to consume you, the longer it will take to reach your destiny. This journey is about no one but you. The longer you doubt your ability to DO you stand in the way of GOD. I remember having to teach soldiers. I had never taught in front of more than five people before so I thought of everything that could go wrong. I had diarrhea, started sweating, would lose focus and l lost the crowd. They listened but my evaluations were a reflection of my fear. There are no set guidelines to accomplishing a goal. Everyone does it differently and they move at a speed that fits their lifestyle. Go at your pace, find what works and move. Don't allow fear to stop you! Be BOLD, CONFIDENT, and have FAITH because its about you and GOD, not you and the world.

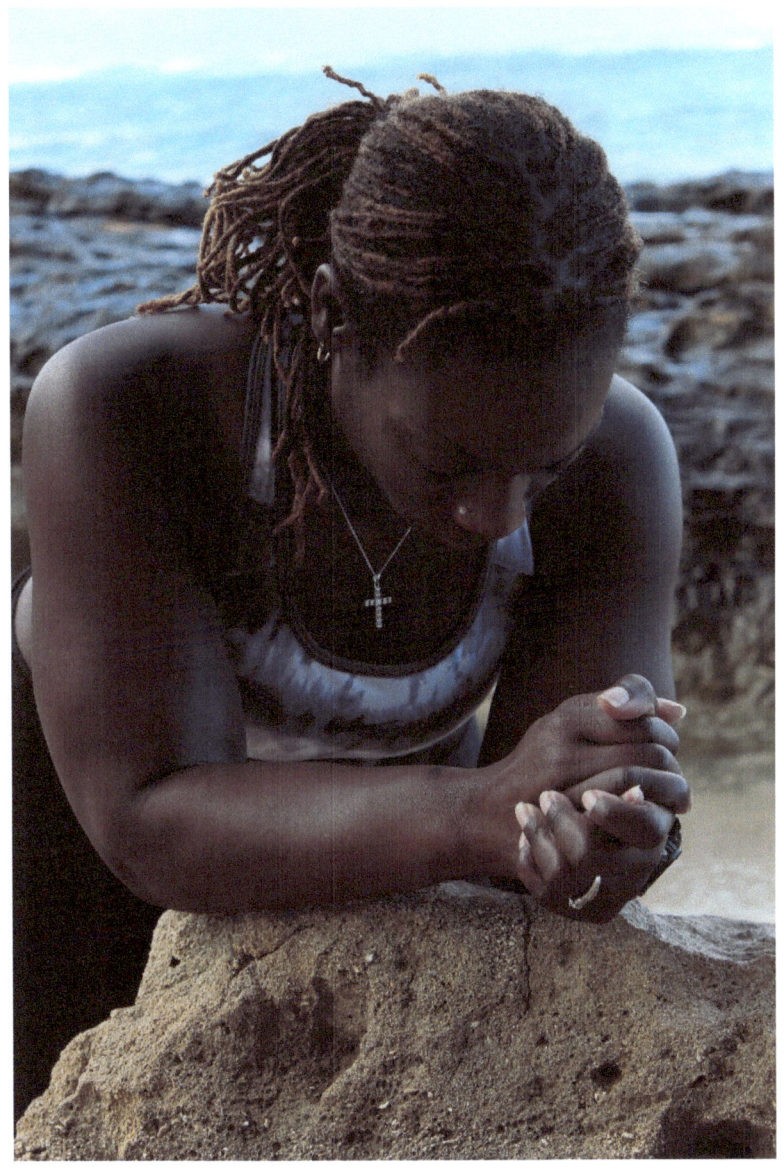

Journal Notes:

Do you have faith in your goals?

Why or Why not?

_____

_____

_____

_____

_____

_____

_____

_____

_____

_____

_____

_____

_____

_____

DAY 11

Change is good

Our decisions are usually based on how we view ourselves or how others view us. The decisions we make are internal motivators, but they are not always clear. Those decisions can be like a clear glass of water or a glass of brown dirty water filled with problems from the world and/or issues of the heart. Making a decision to live a healthy lifestyle is not easy because you think you are going to be missing out on pleasure but in reality the pleasures you will be inheriting are far more rewarding.

~ THE ROAD TO HEALTH OPENS THE DOOR TO MANY OPPORTUNITIES

Journal Notes:

Since you have made the change to live healthier, how has it been? What things have changed? What are you still working on?

_____

_____

_____

_____

_____

_____

_____

_____

_____

_____

_____

_____

_____

_____

_____

_____

_____

_____

DAY 12

Where is your mind?

Just because you made a decision to lose weight doesn't mean everything is going to flow easily. The things of the world have gotten us in the state of unhealthiness. In order for health to be our main event, we will have to look up to a greater source of help. The bible states, *"If then you were raised with Christ, seek those things which are, above where Christ is, sitting at the right hand of God. Set your mind on things above, not on things on the earth." Col 3:1-2*

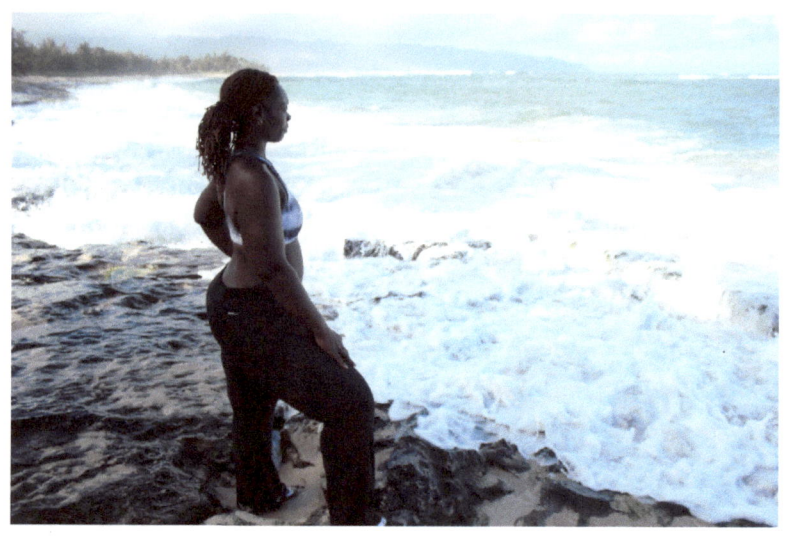

Journal Notes:

What are some ways you can stay focused on your journey?

_____

_____

_____

_____

_____

_____

_____

DAY 13

Got Goals?

"For I know the plans I have for you, declares the Lord, plans to prosper you and not harm you, plans to give you hope and a future." Jeremiah 29:11

Have you ever sat quietly and allowed your mind to just have fun walking around? It could be very mind boggling. Other times you sit and dream about this or dream about that. The dream in your heart will only be a dream if you keep wishing and never doing something to make your dream a reality. Most see themselves healthy yet they do not write out the steps needed to get there. In order for goals to manifest we must be SMART. S.M.A.R.T. is specific, measurable, attainable, realistic and timely. The goals you make are the keys to living boldly, confident and fearless.

~ Put your goal into action

Journal Notes:

Write your goals out and use the S.M.A.R.T. tool

_____

_____

_____

_____

_____

_____

_____

_____

_____

_____

_____

_____

_____

_____

_____

_____

_____

_____

DAY 14
Whose beat are you following?

Are you marching to the beat of someone else's drum? An army of soldiers all line up and march in cadence. They have to stay on beat and make sure they hit the right step or they will throw the whole group off. There is always one that just can't get it together because the beat they are following is not their own. You can not follow someone else's foot steps and hope that you get the same result. You will have to step out in order to find out what beat you are suppose to be marching to.

~CHOOSE TO BE DIFFERENT

Journal Notes:

What makes you different from everyone else?

_____

_____

_____

_____

_____

_____

_____

_____

_____

_____

_____

_____

_____

_____

_____

_____

_____

_____

_____

_____

DAY 15

Decisions, Decisions, and more Decisions

"When you sow, you do not plant the body that will be, but just a seed, perhaps of wheat or of something else." *1 Cor. 15:37*

When we decide to do something we usually try to go ahead in our minds and figure out the outcome before it is manifest. However, those perceived manifestations set us up for failure. Have you ever planned something and it didn't work out the way you imagined it would? This causes disappointment and anger, and we begin to see a distorted view of ourselves. We then start saying things like, "I never will," "I can not," and "why even bother." Seeds of greatness takes time to grow. You did not gain the weight overnight so stop predicting it will fall off in 30, 60, and 90 days. Sow your seeds and watch your plant grow into beauty and brightness.

~ SLOW IS THE NEW FAST

Journal Notes:

What seeds are you sowing?

_____

_____

_____

_____

_____

_____

_____

_____

_____

_____

_____

_____

_____

_____

_____

_____

_____

_____

_____

DAY 16

Feed Me

3 The tempter came to him and said, " If you are the Son of God, tell these stones to become bread." 4 Jesus answered, "It is written, 'Man shall not live on bread alone, but on every word that comes from the mouth of God.' " Matthew 4:3-4

We are bombarded everyday with toxic information from the media, work, friends, and family. Other times we sow seeds of negativity through our thoughts based on what our physical eyes see. Do you take time to empty the garbage? If the trash can is full and we keep putting more trash in it eventually it will spill over. Stop allowing people to deposit their trash in your trash can.

~ CHOOSE TO LIVE OFF PRODUCE AND NOT PROCESSED FOODS

Journal Notes:

What trash do you need to empty today?

_____

_____

_____

_____

_____

_____

_____

_____

_____

_____

_____

_____

_____

_____

_____

_____

_____

_____

_____

DAY 17

Where is your focus?

Are you focused on losing weight or becoming a healthier person? You may think they are the same thing but they are different. When we are focused on losing weight, our focus isn't on how to keep it off. Our focus is I need to lose 30 lbs by this time. When we focus on the physical we base our progress on what we see, which causes distorted views of self. No matter how much weight you lose, you will never be totally satisfied with self. When we make a decision to become a healthier person we must tackle all three dimensions of health; mind, body, and spirit. These three dimensions will keep us stable during our healthy journey. You will learn more about yourself and you are able to figure out what works and what doesn't. This three fold ministry works as a team to help you reach your goal.

~ A healthy lifestyle is a mental activity that resonates outwardly

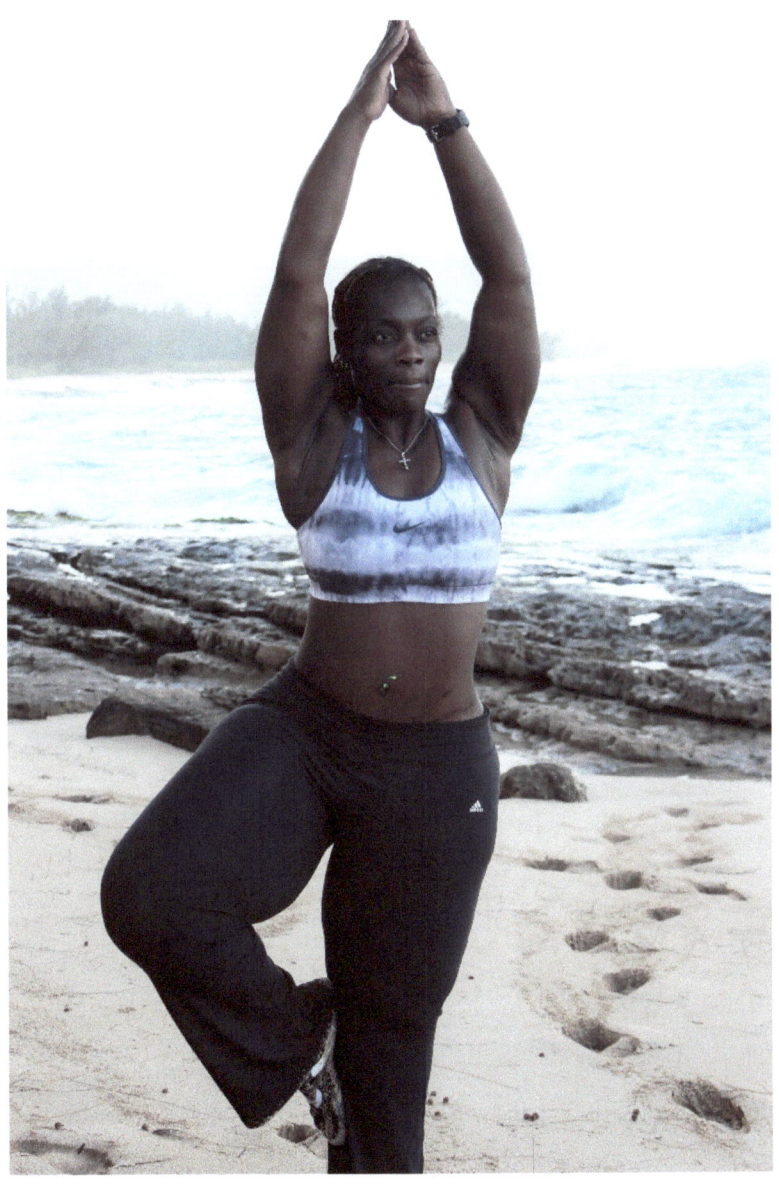

Journal Notes:

What mental challenges are you dealing with on your healthy journey?

_____

_____

_____

_____

_____

_____

_____

_____

_____

_____

_____

_____

_____

_____

_____

_____

_____

_____

_____

_____

_____

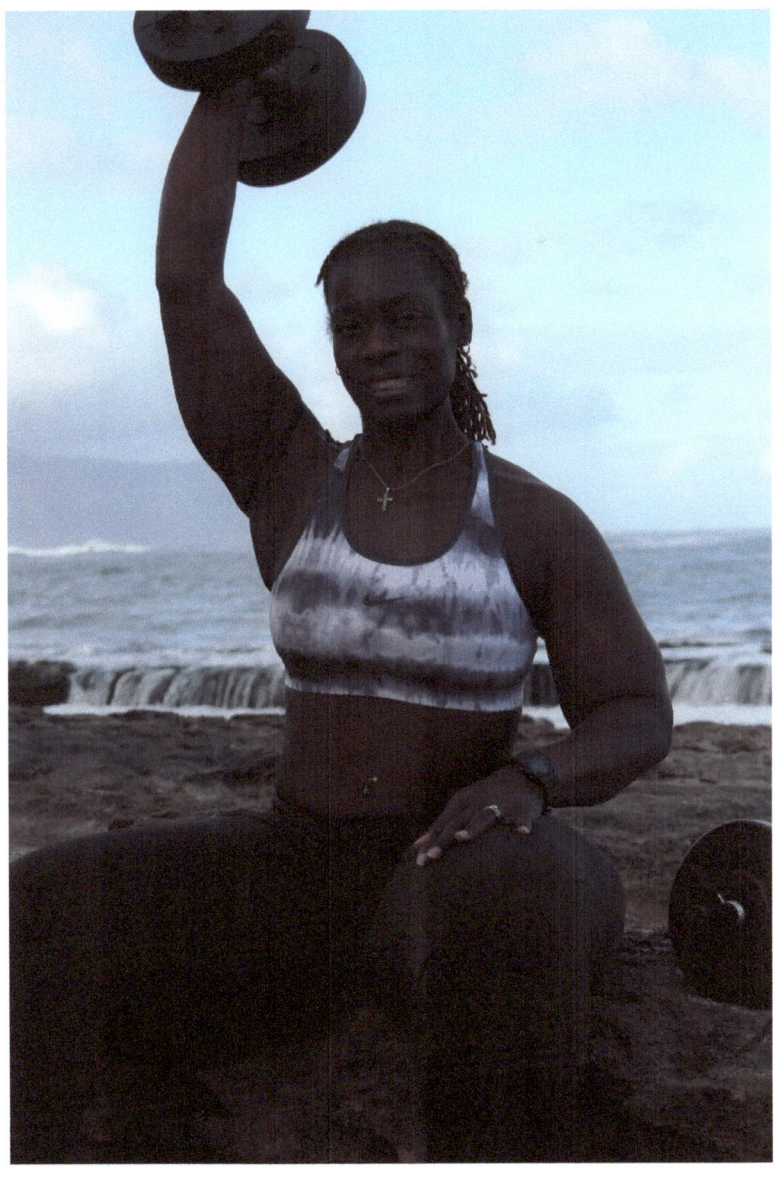

DAY 18

One step at a time

"...he who began a good work in you will carry it on to completion until the day of Christ Jesus." (Philippians 1:6)

I can remember my weight loss journey like it was yesterday. I started out not knowing what to expect because I went in blind. I had good days and bad days. Some were hard and some were easy but I didn't quit. The desire you have in your heart didn't just appear, it was planted there by God because he knew you were capable of succeeding. He knows your end before your beginning. We fall many times but get back up with renewed confidence and keep moving.

~ You win even when you fall

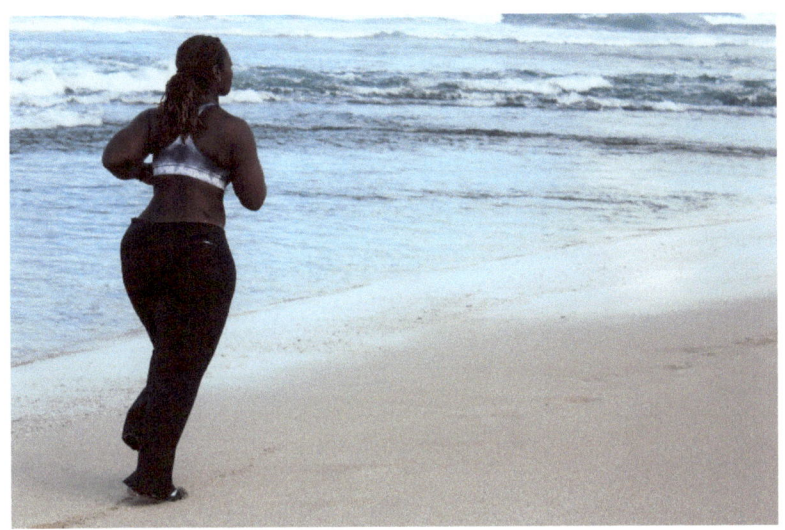

Journal Notes:

What setbacks have you encountered and how did you redeem yourself?

_____

_____

_____

_____

_____

_____

_____

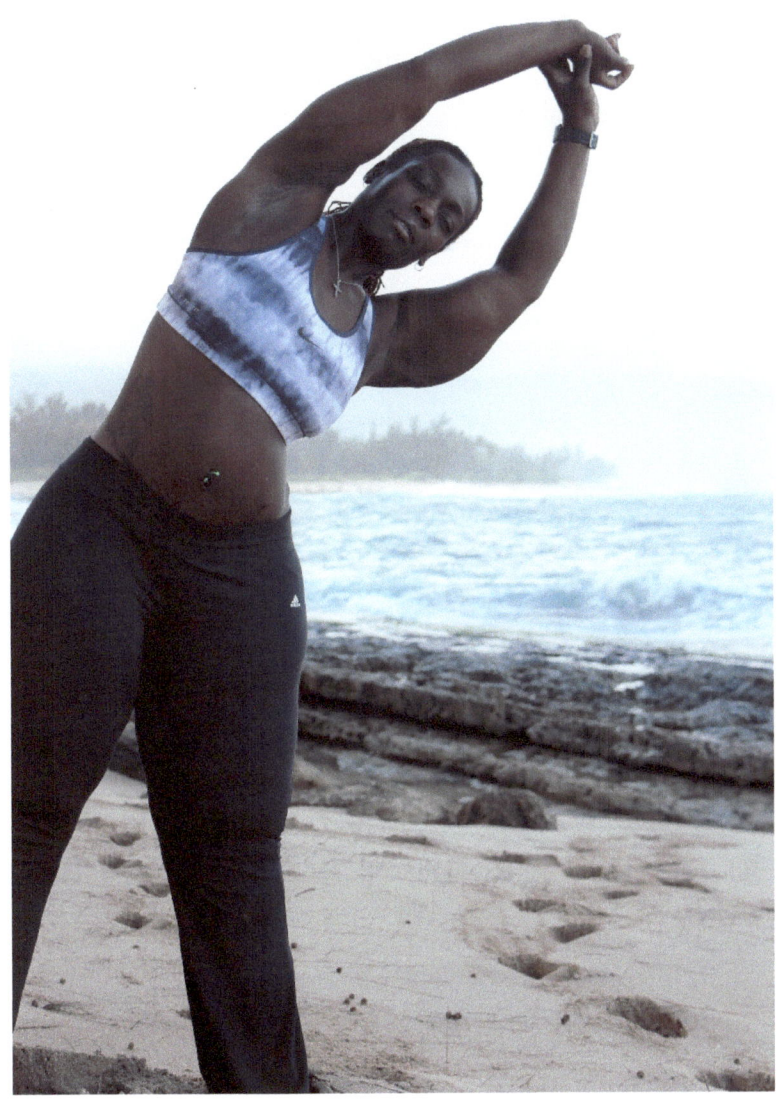

DAY 19

The Eyesight Fight

He replied, "Whether he is a sinner or not, I don't know. I was blind but now I see!" (John 9:25)

Learning to trust when you don't see your way is very hard to do. You don't know what to expect or how to proceed so you literally take it one baby step at a time. Fortunately those baby steps lead to bigger steps and you gain insight on what works and what doesn't. This is what living a healthy lifestyle is all about. Your health is very important but it doesn't initially come easy. You will get mad because you don't have an inkling of how, what, when, where and why you should be eating or doing certain things. The only way I was able to get through it was by reading, praying and meditating. I began to learn things about myself which provided the road map to my success. God knows what you need and He can show you how to get there. Remember the spirit is willing but the flesh is weak.

~ Faith it til you make it

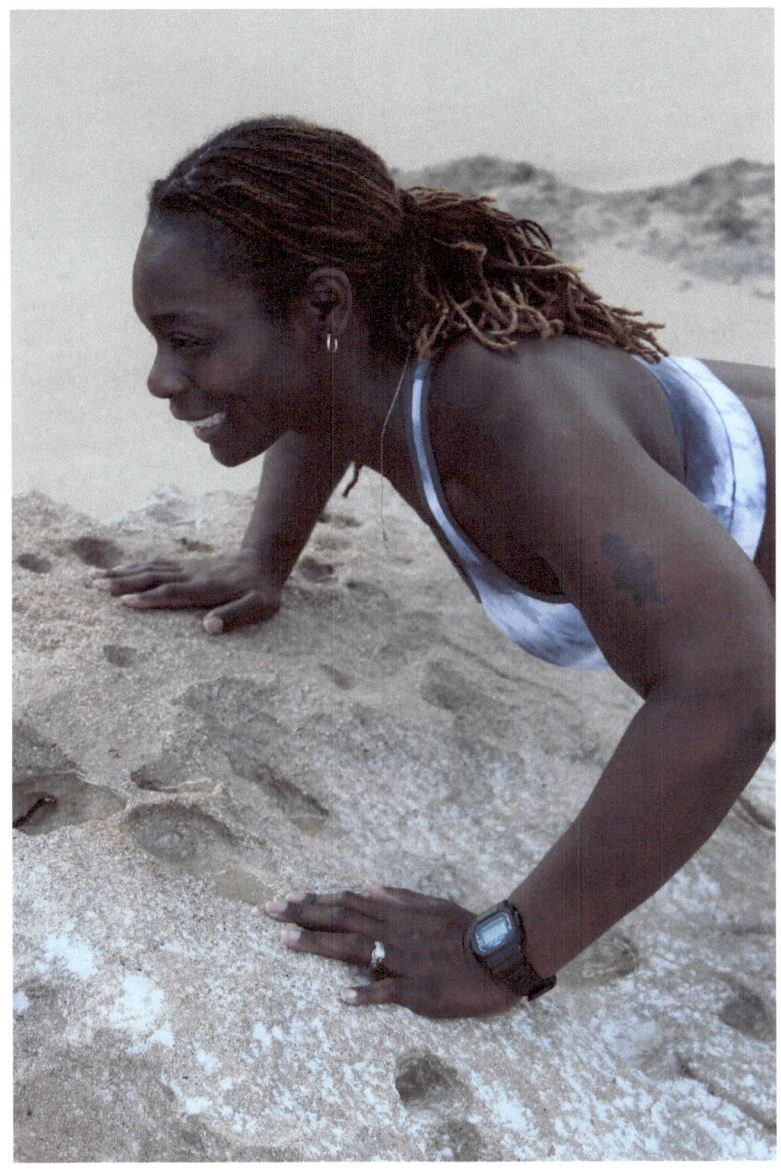

Journal Notes:

Your plan is not always, God's plan. What have you discovered about yourself?

_____

_____

_____

_____

_____

_____

_____

_____

_____

_____

_____

_____

_____

_____

_____

_____

_____

_____

_____

_____

DAY 20
Road map to Success

"May he give you the desire of your heart and make all your plans succeed." (Psalm 20:4)

The plan God has for your life has been written and there is nothing you can do to rewrite it. When we try to do things on our own, the plans God has for you are delayed but never denied. God had a plan for the children of Israel, yet they could not get it together so they delayed God's plan. It is never fun having to do something over and over again because of your disobedience to God, yourself and others who may be involved. Being healthy means you are free of ailments. God desires for you to be healthy and you will get there by walking it out and staying focused. I don't know about you, but I don't want a 6-9 month journey to take 40 years!

~ JESUS TAKE THE WHEEL

Journal Notes:

What does your road map look like? Is it self driven or God driven?

_____

_____

_____

_____

_____

_____

_____

_____

_____

_____

_____

_____

_____

_____

_____

_____

_____

_____

DAY 21

DO YOU BELIEVE?

"Therefore I say to you, whatever things you ask when you pray, believe that you receive them and you will have them."
Matthew 11:24

Life is a puzzle and many times we find ourselves stuck trying to figure out which piece goes where. Notice that when we think we can do it on our own, it makes it just that much harder to find the piece that fits. Deciding to live a healthier lifestyle is just like putting a puzzle together. Having to find what exercise works for your body, what to eat and when to eat can be tedious at times, but its at this moment you will have to draw in and seek help from God. Just as God helped Meshach, Shadrach, and Abednego He can help you. Don't give up because it has gotten hard or you have fallen. The Bible states, " a righteous man falls seven times and rises again, but the wicked are overthrown by calamity (Proverbs 24:16)." Keep climbing til you reach the top.

~ Trust the process

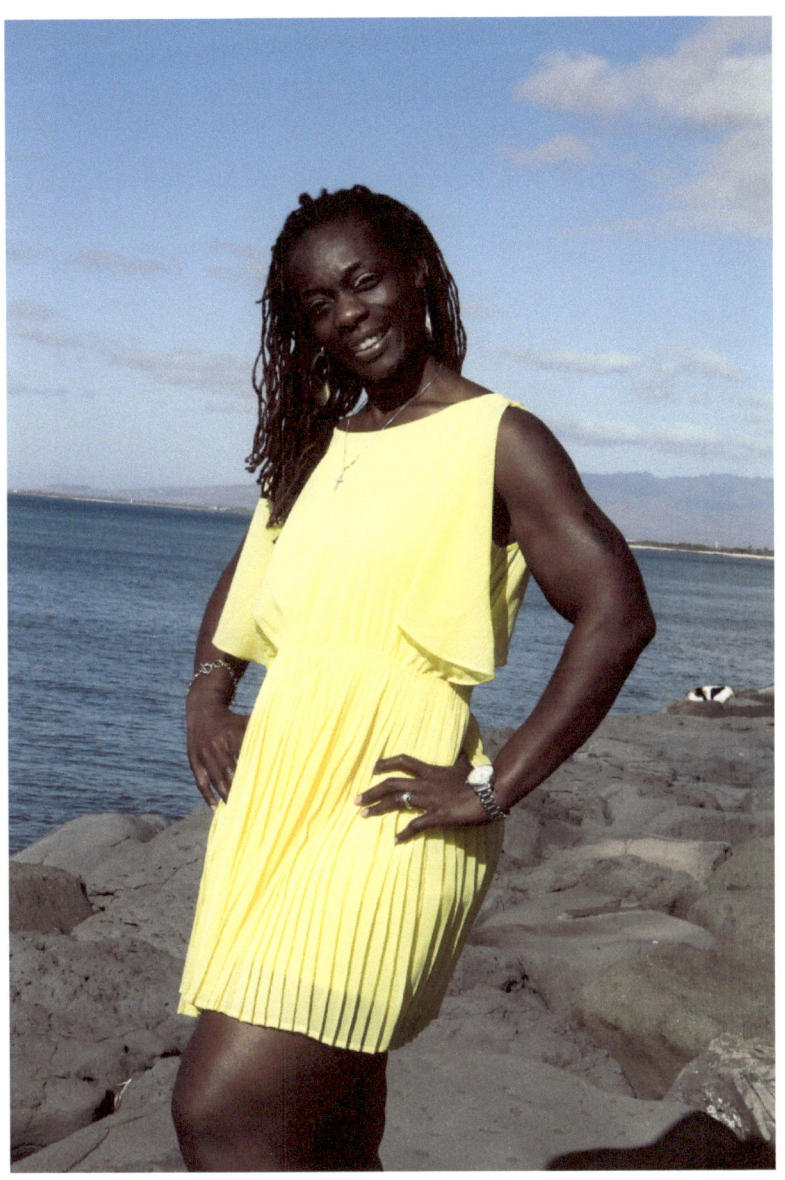

Journal Notes:

It takes 21 days to form a habit, what habits have you formed since learning how to live a Size Healthy Lifestyle?

_____

_____

_____

_____

_____

_____

_____

_____

_____

_____

_____

_____

_____

_____

_____

_____

_____

_____

_____

_____

_____

_____

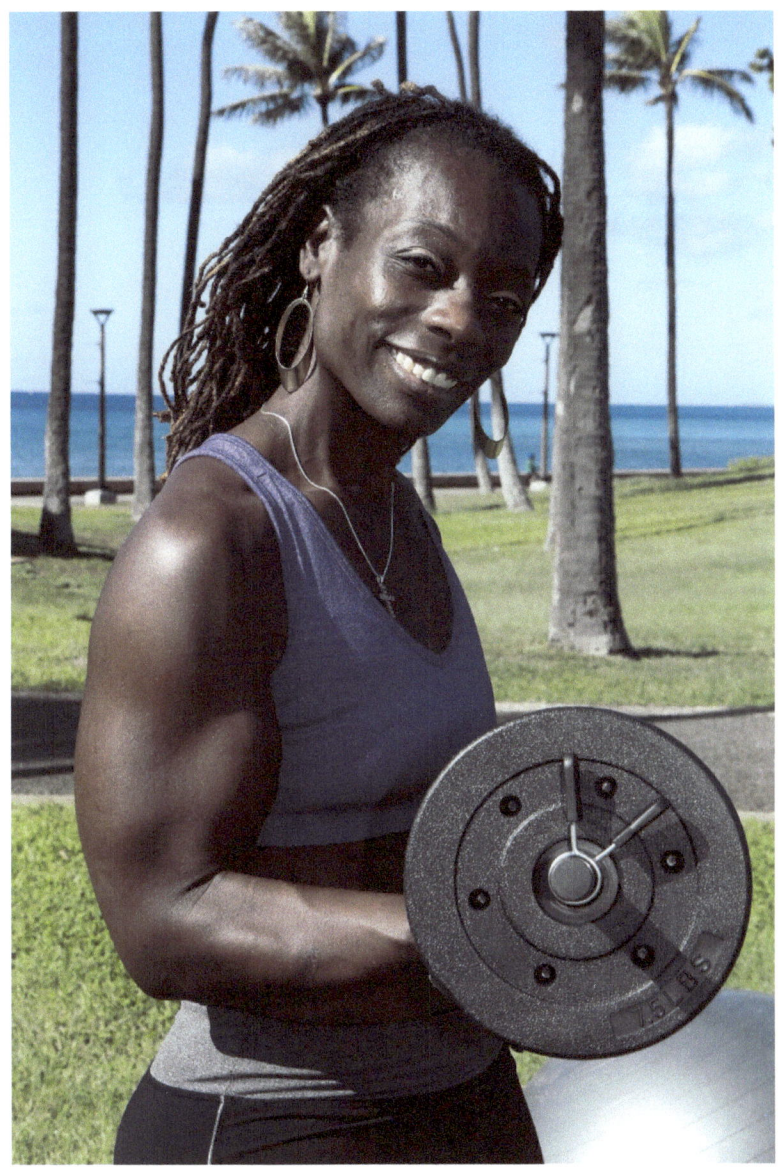

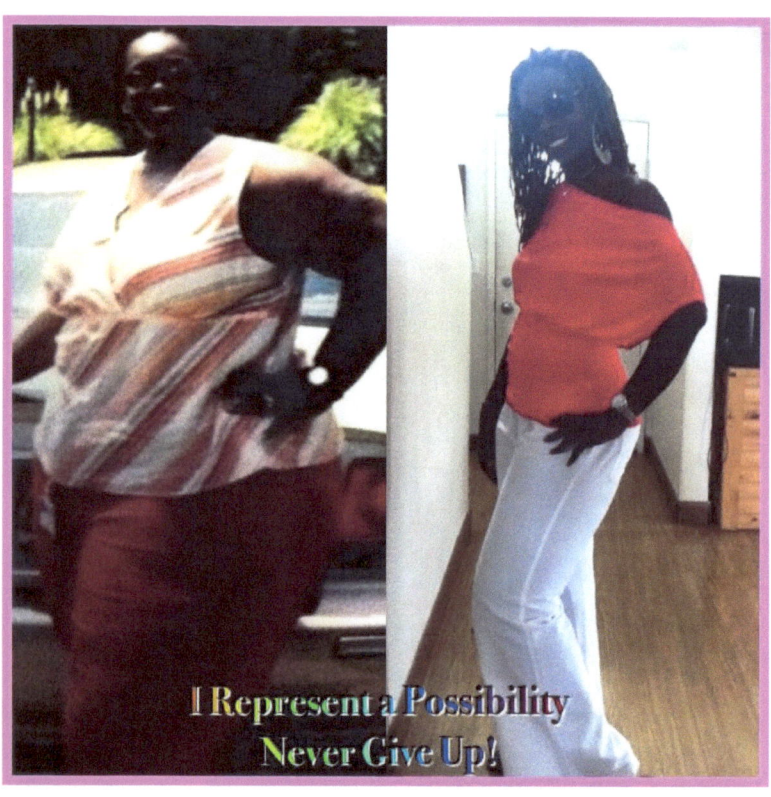

It has taken me seven years to lay aside the mental, physical and spiritual weight. In those seven years, I fell many times before reaching my destination. If I can leave you with one thing, it would be to NEVER GIVE UP. You may have 10 lbs, 30 lbs, or even 100 lbs to lose but know its not the physical imperfections that hold you back. It is your mind that tells you you can't do it, your not good enough, and your dream will never come to past. This is where the work lies in conquering your unhealthy habits. Everyday you are given another opportunity to work on you. THANK GOD! When things seem to be falling apart, focus on the positives and make positive affirmations about yourself. If you can't find one, let me give you one. If you are reading this you are blessed with eyesight and that alone is something to be thankful for. No situation is too hard for God, but you must believe that HELP is on its way.

I represent a possibility so if I can do it, so can you.

YOUniquely Designed,

Nataisha "ADivaRunner" Ramirez

Founder/CEO Size Healthy LLC

www.ingramcontent.com/pod-product-compliance
Lightning Source LLC
Chambersburg PA
CBHW050807290526

45792CB00001B/20